# Caregiving with Laughter
## A Husband's Perspective

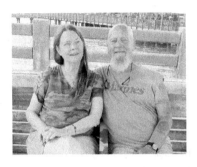

## "Mr. Steve" Adzima

Anabella
St. Augustine, FL

Book design by Sagaponack Books & Design
Photographs by Stephen Adzima
Poem by Jim Hatcher used with permission from the author

ISBNs:
978-1-7375995-0-0 (softcover)
978-1-7375995-1-7 (hardcover)
978-1-7375995-2-4 (e-book)

Library of Congress Catalog Card Number: 2021918516

Summary: A husband's personal vignettes on finding laughter in the serious job of being a caregiver for a spouse with Alzheimer's disease.

HEA039140 Health & Fitness / Diseases / Alzheimer's & Dementia
HEA028000 Health & Fitness / Health Care Issues
BIO026000 Biography & Autobiography / Personal Memoirs

First Edition
Printed in the USA

This book is dedicated to Susana and Phyllis, the loves of my life, and to all the caregivers out there. May your journey in caregiving be as blessed as mine has—filled with love, understanding, and laughter.

*Laughter is, and always will be,*
*the best form of therapy.*

—Dau Voire

# Table of Contents

# Introduction

Let me take this page to introduce you to Susana, my late wife, and Phyllis, my current wife. Susana started out with breast cancer, then proceeded to ovarian cancer. This is when I started being a caregiver.

Next came Phyllis, my current wife, who has Alzheimer's. In the book you will see: how I dealt with these tragedies, the way my mind thinks, and the things I came up with to cope with the ever changing conditions of my wives; what might be coming your way; and, hopefully, some suggestions that might help.

Be open minded and be resourceful! You may even see why I call it Funheimer's instead of Alzheimer's, and caretaker instead of caregiver. I believe all caregivers are very special and chosen to be caregivers. Bless all of you!

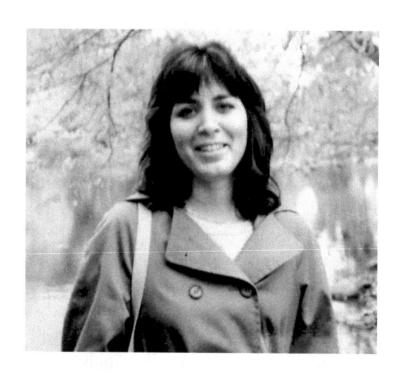

her laugh, if only for a short while. I still have a shaved head to this day.

There was nothing I wouldn't do for her. Whatever I could do for her, I would do. As time went on (two plus years), she became weaker and weaker. We only had one bathroom in the house, and she wasn't able to get up the stairs anymore. (I didn't know anything about hospice at the time, so I handled everything myself.) I made a small toilet box out of plywood so she could go on the first floor; then I could slide out the container and take it upstairs to the bathroom to empty it.

Susana loved to go for rides; I would take her anywhere I could think of or she could suggest. Whatever it took to make her happy, I would try to do.

I always assured her everything would be all right. (Always reassuring and being positive.) In my heart I felt she knew she wasn't winning the battle. Sometimes when we were out riding, I would see her looking at people. I asked her what she was looking for. She said she was looking for someone for me to be with when she wasn't around anymore.

Eventually, between Christmas and New Year's, she passed away.

She was an awesome lady who would do anything for her two daughters (my stepdaughters). She is deeply missed and loved.

God bless my Susana.

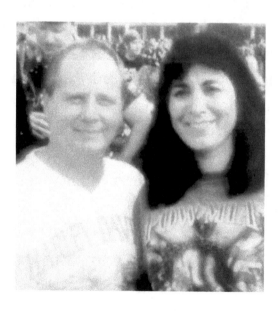

# The Susana and Phyllis Connection

*I*n our New Jersey community, the pastor at the Ellisdale Church also pastors at the Crosswicks Church four miles away. I was unaware that the pastor had mentioned Sue at the Crosswicks Church where Phyllis attended. He mentioned how sick she was and that I was taking good care of her.

One day, Sue received a letter from Phyllis, saying she was sorry for her illness and to let her know if she could do anything for her.

I know in my heart that the Lord put both Susana and Phyllis in my life so I could take care of them.

I knew Phyllis from the third grade (1953). We went all through grammar school and high school together, but we didn't hang with the same people. It was not until Susana was sick and received the letter from Phyllis, that I even remembered or thought of Phyllis.

About seven weeks after Susana went to the Lord, I took myself to a movie. After the movie I was going to leave the mall, but something stopped me and told me to walk through the mall.

So I did. I had my head shaved, with an earring in my ear, and a heavy flannel shirt on. As I got to the second floor, I saw Phyllis walking toward me. She wouldn't look at me. (Later she told me I looked scary and maybe like a stabber.) As she walked by, I said, "Phyllis." She stopped and turned around. She said she recognized my voice. (I was probably just too handsome to resist!) We talked for a minute and we went to the first floor, where we sat and drank Pepsi and talked for four hours.

After a number of years seeing each other, we were married on the back sun porch of Phyllis's house (in New Jersey), by our favorite pastor.

The rest is all history.

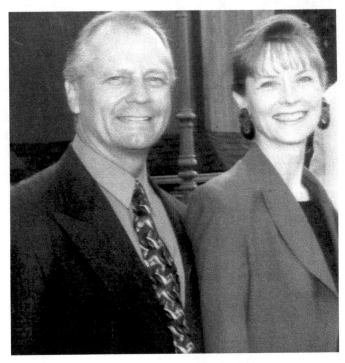

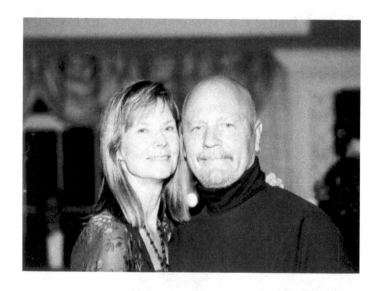

# Then Came My Phyllis: Twelve Years Now

Phyllis first started to show signs of memory loss twelve years ago. She was a volunteer at the library. We only lived across the street from the library, but I always wanted her to drive the car there because I felt it was safer.

One day she came home from volunteering, and I asked her where the car was.

Her answer was that she didn't know. I said, "Did you leave it at the library?" Again she said, "I don't know." She had completely forgotten that she had driven there.

I said, "Let's go take a walk over to the parking lot and see if it's there." (I was hoping no one had stolen the car.) Sure enough, it was there. At that point, I started paying more attention to what was going on. Very slowly, things started going downhill. Everyone goes down at a different rate.

One time I went to the gym. I told her numerous times where I was going. She started to panic, not knowing where I was. She called me eight times, but I hadn't taken my phone to the gym. When I arrived back home, she was extremely relieved.

I started putting pieces of paper taped to the door or wall, wherever I thought she couldn't possibly miss them, telling her where I was and when I thought I would be home.

It worked for a while. Then she started not seeing them.

Next thing I did was purchase a dry erase board. I installed it near the back door and where the car keys were hung, right near the kitchen. I would write the current date, time I left, time to come home, and where I was going. That was a good move and worked well for a period of time. I have recommended that to many people, and it has worked well for them also.

At times we would fly from Florida to the Northeast to visit relatives. When we arrived at the airport, sometimes she would ask who we were waiting for. She didn't recall that we were the people flying. She would want to know where we were going.

I would tell her as many times as she asked— whatever she needed to be comfortable.

This is where REASSURANCE comes in. Let them know everything is all right. Watch their face and see it relax, and know the whole body relaxes and stays relaxed for a while with the reassurance.

This was okay for a few years. Then she would start getting confused, not knowing where she was.

I decided that I would need to stay in one place for her to be comfortable, so we sold the house that we still owned up north and stayed in Florida.

# The Hurricane Incident

The day before Hurricane Matthew, my 96-year-old mother was in the hospital for a procedure. She gave me a call in the morning, saying they were not going to do the procedure. Something with her heart rate? We live just over the bridge from the hospital, so my wife and I were at the hospital in about fifteen minutes. When we got to my mother's room, about four people were there, ready to stick her with needles to draw more blood. I walked in and said, "No blood draw if you're not going to do the procedure. You're not going to take more blood!"

I told them to get the paperwork ready because I was taking her home. We took my mother home, to her house, and spent the night with her. That night the hurricane came. Everything is electric, and we lost power. The temperature was in the 90s the next day, with no AC and a weak 96-year-old.

The rain stopped, and Mom asked if we could at least put some chairs outside and have some breeze. I said "Sure," and set up three chairs. (Keep in mind we could not get home because they had closed the bridge.) Mom sat in a chair, and I started to sit next to her, when a yellow jacket hornet came out of nowhere and stung me. (I am highly allergic to yellow jackets. My wife has saved me twelve times with EPI pens!) Phyllis shot me with an EPI pen, and I called 911. The ambulance came and I had to decide whether to take

Phyllis with me to the hospital or leave her with my weakened mother. I decided to leave her with Mom.

I was rushed to the hospital with all the IVs and medication. They kept me there for a few hours till I was stabilized, and then I was released. Now, how do I get back to Mom's? No vehicles were on the road. No taxis were running. All the people I could have called lived on the other side of the bridge. I was "shit out of luck"! I knew I needed to get back to take care of Mom and Phyllis. My cell phone was down to 7 percent.

So, this is where the Dynamic Duo comes in. I give them a call. Remember, Mom is too weak to drive and Phyllis doesn't know where to go. She has lost all sense of direction due to Alzheimer's. I have run out of options. I asked Mom if she could get in the passenger side of the car. She said yes. I asked Phyllis if she could drive if my mother told her where to go. She said yes.

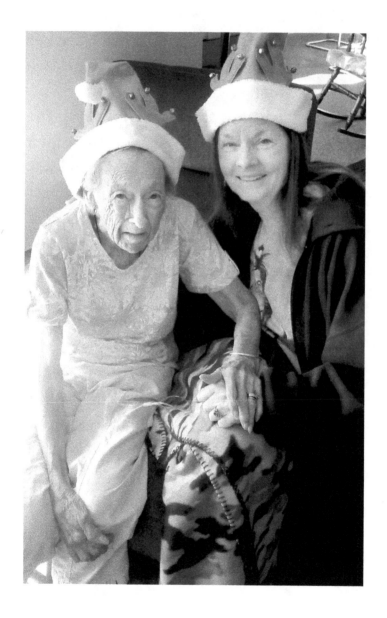

So, now I thought I was in good hands. Cell phone is now down to 4 percent. Nobody has come for me. I receive a call. They can't get the car started and I can hear the car beeping in the background. So I go through all the steps with the remote, to reset the alarm and how to start the car, and asked them to call me before they left. I never heard from them again. They forgot to call me. I left the hospital and started walking down Route 1. Ten minutes later I could see them coming down the road. A welcome sight! I got behind the wheel, went back to Mom's, and cooked dinner for us on our Coleman camping stove.

The following day the bridge reopened and we could take Mom back to our house, where we had power and AC. What a Dynamic Duo— Mom and Phyllis!

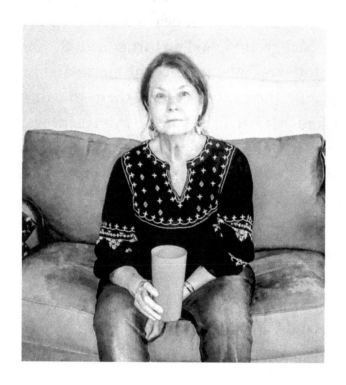

# Not Knowing Me

The other evening while riding home from town, Phyllis asked me how she was going to get home. That is when I knew she was starting a new level of memory loss.

I said that I was taking her home, and I asked her if she knew who I was. She didn't know and called me someone else. After asking her a series of questions to see what she did and did not remember, I told her my name, that we were married, and we were going home to our house where just she and I live.

She seemed reassured.

The next day it happened again. This time she thought I was her cousin. Again I told her who I was and reassured her. It calmed her down. I am aware that it will happen more often. It bothered me for about a day. Then I decided that I could be anyone she thought I was! It would be better for her to keep her calm and happy.

It's better to accept it than to correct her. It would only frustrate your loved one.

And I can be whoever I need to be. The key is to accept it and know that you are not going to change anything.

It happened again, while coming home from a ride over to Vilano Beach in the evening. On the way back, Phyllis said, "I don't have anywhere to go. Who will take care of me?" I knew at that point she was completely lost and felt there was nothing around for her.

I immediately pulled over to remind and reassure her that I was always going to take care of her, that we were married, and we were on our way home.

She immediately threw her arms around me, started kissing me and kept thanking me. She was relieved and then started to get back to normal. After I got her home and gave her a tour of the house, everything was good again.

## Reassured Again

One evening I noticed Phyllis just didn't seem right. I asked if something was bothering her. She said that she was all right. Things didn't seem to be getting any better, so I asked her again.

She wasn't able to find the words, but she said, "A long time ago." I asked, but she couldn't find any words to tell me what was wrong. I asked if someone had done something bad to her or hurt her, but she couldn't say. I couldn't find out anything else.

So I looked at her and told her whatever had happened was in the past, and nothing was going to harm her now. I reassured her everything was okay. She stepped toward me, put her arms around me, and very emotionally kept thanking me over and over.

All it took was reassurance to make everything okay again.

Reassurance is so important!

# The Shower

We loved living on Nelmar Avenue. We never wanted to live anywhere else.

But one day while we were out riding, we took a right onto what looked like a dirt road. All of a sudden there was this secret housing development I had no idea was there. While driving through the development, we saw a house for sale. It had been on the market for four days. I called my friend (a realtor) and told him I wanted to see it right away. We were in it two hours later.

The first thing I noticed (other than Phyllis's eyes bulging) was the main bathroom. It was all tiled and wheelchair accessible. The shower was also wheelchair accessible, with no step into the shower. There was a built-in seat. (I call it a 2½-ass seat.) I was sold! Simply because of the shower and feeling we would need the accessibility one day. I didn't even notice it backed up to a beautiful saltwater marsh.

About a month later we were in the house.

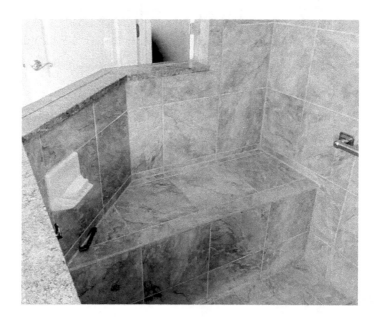

It happened just at the right time. The first week we moved in, Phyllis started to need help taking a shower. At first it was just directions on what to do. Then, as time went on, she needed more and more help, not remembering how to wash and then not knowing how to rinse. But, as I always like to do, HAVE FUN, MAKE HER LAUGH.

Her whole body would relax as she was laughing.

Here is what I did: I told her we were going to make believe she was a car at the car wash, and was getting the Admiral Treatment at the Showboat Car Wash. Her face was the grille, her arms were front fenders, and her legs were rear fenders. Her breasts were headlights, her butt (or ass) is where the exhaust comes out, and I will leave it to your imagination where the dipstick went. I would talk her through the whole car wash, and she would laugh throughout the whole wash-and-rinse cycle. I highly recommend the car wash!

The other event in the bathroom is the Olympic Panty Toss. Put her panties on her right foot and kick them across the room, trying to get them in the dirty clothes hamper. (We make it a competition and I do my underpants.) WE BOTH LAUGH THE WHOLE TIME! As their brain changes and regresses, they don't like to have water on their face (like a child). I now use the handheld shower attachment. It works much better. I also put a ten-foot extension on the handheld; gives more flexibility. It was about $12.00 on the internet. She loves the handheld.

One other note: For shampoos, use 2-in-1 shampoo and conditioner; makes it easier for you.

I also recommend Ivory soap, because it rinses very easily.

One last event in the shower: I would wait until her eyes were closed, and I would put on glasses with a mustache attached (from the Dollar Store). Only problem I had was that when it got wet, the black mustache would fall off and get all over the shower. But it was worth it to see her laugh!

## Additions for Taking a Shower

Play Simon Says:

> Simon says: Raise your arms.
> Simon says: Close your eyes.
> Simon says: Open your legs.
> Simon says: Bend over.

And, of course, you add some comments that Simon doesn't say.

This way, taking a shower is fun! You laugh and everyone gets clean.

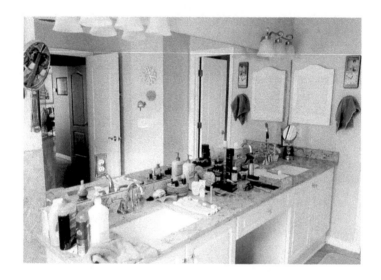

# Reflections

People's minds deteriorate at different rates.

One thing to watch out for is a problem with reflections.

Our house is all sliding glass doors on the rear. We also have many mirrors throughout the house. My wife will become very confused looking in the mirror, thinking someone else is there. At times, in the bathroom I have offered her a tissue, and she reached her hand out, crashing into the mirror, thinking the tissue was there.

I am not sure what I am going to do about the bathroom mirror; maybe hang a valance or some removable decals. She also looks through the shower glass, sees her own image, and thinks someone is there.

In the front room, I have switched where she sits, so that her back is to the mirror. As for the sliding glass doors, I have decided not to wash them. It cuts down on the reflections.

I have now covered the nine-foot mirror in the bathroom. Phyllis had been talking to herself and laughing and having a good time. I asked her what was going on. She said, "We were just laughing." (Her and her image.) I said, "Great! Glad you are having a good time. Both of you, come into the other room with me." (I didn't want a crowd of people in the house!) I finally decided to cover the bathroom mirror with a "custom-designed drape."

I picked up a discounted piece of fabric from Walmart, five grommets, and five S-hooks.

And there you have a custom designer drape! It seems to be working for the last couple of days. I have also draped towels over the shower glass, and that also stops all the reflections. Tomorrow I'll pick up more custom drapery from Walmart and cover the mirror in the front room.

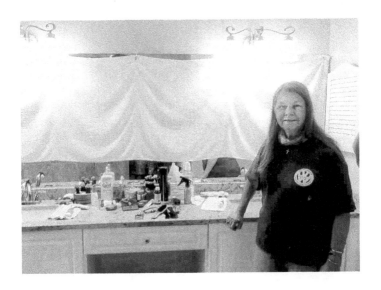

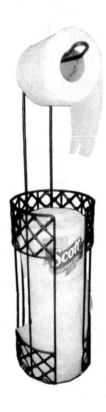

# The Toilet

Phyllis has never had a problem going to the bathroom. Then one day she called me into the toilet room and said she had to poop. I said to go ahead. She sat on the toilet and asked how to go. I told her to sit for a little bit, take her time, and maybe tighten her stomach up and try to get something out.

It worked, and that was the last I heard of it for a while. But I knew it would happen more and more often as her forgetfulness progressed. Now we are at the place where I go to the pot with her to assist with directions. She now can't find the bathroom (at home), so I take her there, wait for her to go, then assist with the wiping with the toilet paper. I distribute it to her. First wipe: wipe and drop; second wipe: wipe and drop; third: wipe and peek. Then we continue until she is clean.

When the job is complete and ready to flush, we stand at attention, salute, I hum "Taps," and we flush the toilet together. Sort of a military send-off. We have fun and she laughs. (I always look for the fun things.) ALWAYS HAVE FUN! One incident that happened to me: We were out driving and all of a sudden I really had to go to the bathroom. We rushed home and I ran through the garage to the bathroom (just making it in time).

After the job was complete, I reached for the toilet paper that wasn't there (only an empty). I knew that in the other bathroom I had four rolls in the dispenser, so I called Phyllis and asked her to get me a roll and bring it to me. She said "Sure," and off she went.

A couple of minutes later she came back and asked me what she was supposed to get. (By now I was laughing so hard I almost fell off the seat.) So I told her and sent her off again. This time she comes back and says she can't find the bathroom.

Then I found a pad and pencil in the bathroom and drew her a map to the other bathroom. She came back and said she couldn't read the map. Now I am really laughing! I ask her to find her cell phone.

Finally she finds it. Now I call her phone with my cell phone and walk her through the house. She brings back the toilet paper, and we laugh all day. Later that day we bought another toilet paper dispenser that holds multiple rolls.

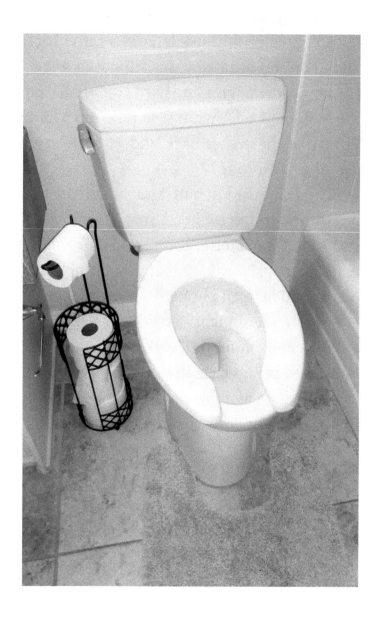

# The Recycle Incident

We came home from a ride because Phyllis had to go to the bathroom. I brought her into the house and the bathroom, and asked her what she needed to do. Of course her response was, "I don't know." I told her, "Do what you need to do. I will take the recycles out to the curb, and I'll be right back." I took the recycling out and came back into the house.

There she was sitting on the toilet with her underpants, shorts, and sneakers all off. I asked her what she was doing. She responded: "I don't know." I asked her if she went to the bathroom. She said, "I think so." Then I noticed that the toilet seat lid was down. That was scary, so we now have toilet seats that don't have lids.

Now I started to get her dressed. "No," I said, "you need underpants first, and then the shorts." Then I asked what happened to her underpants liner. She didn't know.

You can imagine that by now we are laughing ourselves silly! So I finally got her dressed in the proper sequence. We laughed all night about what happened. But of course, anytime I mentioned it, it was like it was the first she had heard about it, each time.

It was a fun evening—another example of accepting the situation and making the best of it!

# Television

She is at the point now that she feels that the people on television are also in the room with us. Sometimes she will touch their faces with her hand, or if they are waving on TV, she will start waving back.

The other morning we were watching television before we got out of bed. There were four people on the screen at the same time, one in each corner. I told Phyllis that we needed to get up and start our day. She told me she couldn't get out of bed with all the people in our bedroom.

I have to reassure her all the time that it is just her and me in the house. Then she is okay.

I try to find funny programs for her to watch. That helps keep her relaxed. If we are watching a drama, she thinks it is happening right here to us. Then I have to explain that it's just a TV show. Once I explain it to her, I can see her relax.

# The Straw

As people with Alzheimer's lose their three-dimensional eyesight, they lose the ability to see what is in front of them. Most drinking straws are clear when you go out to eat in a restaurant.

As time goes on, people with Alzheimer's can't see the glass or drink in front of them and the straw becomes invisible. Starbucks is one place that has a colored straw (green). At first I would take straws from Starbucks and use them when I took her to other places.

But now she can't see the straw at all, and it has become very dangerous. One time it stuck in her cheek, another time up her nose, and another time almost in her eye. I now always remove the straw from her glass and mine, so she sees we are doing the same.

On a recent trip to McDonald's in the evening, to treat her to a hot fudge sundae (I am a big spender—nothing but the best!), we sat in the car to eat.

She suddenly said to me, "Nothing is coming out." I looked over and she was trying to suck through the spoon that was in the ice cream. I told her it was a spoon, not a straw. She started to eat the ice cream after I demonstrated how to use the spoon. But, once again, she said something was wrong.

I looked over and she was trying to use the spoon as a straw again. I gave her another lesson and helped her with the next couple of bites. I told her it was because the spoons were the color black and hard to see while we were eating in the car, and it wasn't a big deal. We laughed and continued eating.

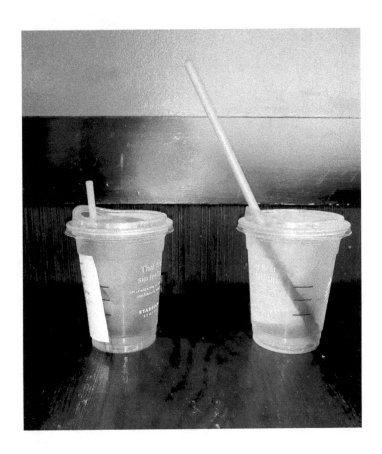

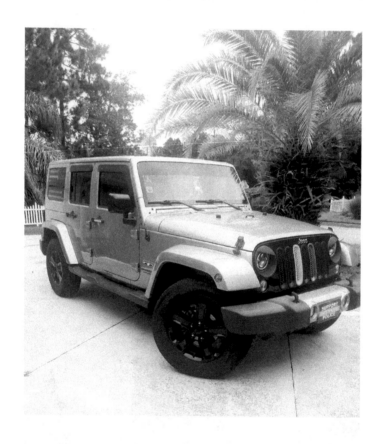

# The Car Door

*T*onight we stopped at the CVS drug
store. I got out of the car. Phyllis got
out of her side and stood there. She
had forgotten that fast if she was getting into
the car or getting out.

Just another fun time! We laughed.

Today I was cutting and installing drywall.
I had Phyllis lie down on the couch, and I
covered her with a blanket, put the TV on, and
told her I would be in the garage working with
the drywall. A very short time had passed.
I looked out the garage door and there she

was, walking in the driveway, WITH JUST A SWEATSHIRT AND SNEAKERS ON.

I quickly moved her into the house. I asked her what was going on. She said she couldn't find anyone in the house, so she went outside to find people. She still thinks people live in our home, other than the two of us. I explained to her that we are the only people who live in the house. She was comforted in knowing that. I helped her get dressed the rest of the way. We laughed and then we were off to see the display of Christmas lights in town.

# The Ice Cream Cone

As nightfall comes, we settle in after eating dinner and going to feed the homeless.

We head to the front room to watch some TV. I have to be careful what I put on the television, because my wife (after losing some of her three-dimensional vision) has a tendency to become overly involved with the show that is on. As an example, we were watching an episode of *Law and Order*. The police had stopped a box truck and had said, "Everyone get out!" Phyllis got up quickly from the couch, said "Let's go," and started to put her sneakers on. I had to tell her it was just a TV show.

Another time, we watched the weather and saw they were expecting 17 inches of snow up north. Everyone was advised to go to the store to get supplies, and the elderly were told to seek shelter. She got up and was ready to go to the store. I explained that we live in Florida and that the weather report was for another area.

In addition to these examples, very often at night she will sit up and say, "Okay, I don't want to be here anymore. I want to go home." Then I explain that we are home. This is our house, and no one else lives here.

This is where the ice cream cone comes in. When she starts getting agitated in the evening, I will give her a Nestlé Drumstick. She instantly calms down, and she takes longer to eat that cone than anyone I have ever seen. It just settles her down and she is good pretty much for the rest of the evening. I make sure to give her a cone every night.

# The Jeans

We got up this morning and it looked like it was going to be a nice warm day. I had Phyllis put on her shorts. We had breakfast and went out to do some errands.

After being out for a while I noticed the temp was starting to fall, so we headed home to have her change into long jeans.

After putting them on, she said they were tight. She doesn't wear them that often, so I told her they would stretch and be more comfortable as she wore them for a while.

Not an hour later, I went into the bathroom to help her. That is when I noticed she had put her long jeans on over her shorts. We made an immediate change and laughed quite a bit.

Again, laughing is the key.

Who said Alzheimer's isn't fun?!

# *Acceptance*

*T*his is one BIG JOB: learning to accept that your loved one is going downhill and you can't do anything about it.

Most people have a hard time with acceptance. You want to be able to give them a magic pill, or change their diet and things will be back to normal again.

It's not happening. Nothing is out there yet. We hope someday there will be, but for now, you need to accept.

Some people get very angry that their loved one is not the same. You have to remember they are doing the best they can, and you need to remember to accept that.

They don't mean to ask you so many questions and have to depend on you for everything. You need to accept this and know it is only going to happen more and more.

Acceptance doesn't come easy. You will have to remind yourself all the time.

But again, always remember they are doing the best they can!

# Patience

Boy, did you ever think you would need as much patience as you do! When they throw the Kleenex on the floor or on the countertop; when they use 50 or more rolls of toilet paper a week; when they don't close the cabinet door or don't push the chair back in. Drives you crazy! But remember they are doing the best they can.

Don't make it hard on yourself. Just pick up the Kleenex, get another roll of toilet paper, close the cabinet door, or push the chair in. That way you are not so frustrated. Just pick up the slack. Not a big deal, and you will be much happier.

I find my patience by praying for it. Every night I ask the Lord, if He has any extra patience, send it my way.

# Hurt Physically or Emotionally

What you need to watch out for and make sure of is that your loved one is not hurt physically or mentally; your mind has to be constantly going and your eyes constantly scanning. You're looking for yourself and for your loved one.

As time goes on and they lose more memory, you have to pick up the slack. As they become more confused, they need to be reassured more often. You can see it by looking in their face. Don't let their feelings be hurt. Keep them smiling and laughing.

Physically, you will need to help them more all the time—like getting into bed.

Our bed is a little higher off the floor. Today's mattresses are made so much taller on the sides, that it makes it more of a challenge to get on and off. You might consider a lower frame.

I take her to the bathroom, or she goes on her own but can't find her way back.

On occasion (and it happens more all the time), she doesn't remember how to get back in bed. Now, you are dealing with another adult and they are not lightweight.

Walk them to their side of the bed and help them get in. You don't want them to fall out! Make sure they are far enough on the bed toward the center, so if they turn on their side they won't fall out of bed.

# Pain

As they go downhill, they lose the ability to feel pain when they are hurting. They also lose the ability to know if they are hot or cold.

Learn to read their face. It tells a lot and can help you know when they are hurting. Watch to see if they are bumping into things.

Check their fingernails so they are not too long, so they won't scratch their eye. Make sure that their toenails are not so long that the nails are digging into other toes.

As for hot or cold, use common sense. If you are cold or chilled, they most likely are also. The same for hot. If you are hot, then they probably are also.

Always keep a light jacket or extra shirt around to keep them comfortable.

# Friends

So you think your loved one has a lot of friends?

When they find out your loved one has dementia, Alzheimer's, cancer, or something else—holy cow! What happened to all those friends? Notice how the phone calls start tapering off. No more cards or invitations coming your way for the cookout or party.

That's just the way it is.

I look at friends as the ones who keep up with you, stay in touch, or come over for a visit. The rest aren't friends; they are just acquaintances. Not a big deal. Just remember you have each other.

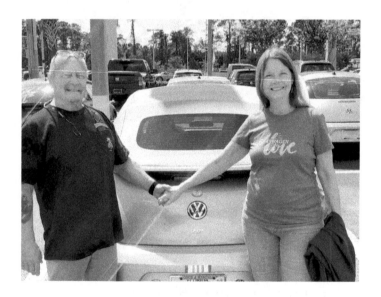

# Sex

The forbidden word. No one mentions sex. Remember your loved one has memory loss, and remember, as natural as sex is, it does require some memory. Don't be surprised if they don't remember how to participate in lovemaking. Don't push the subject. It only makes them upset and uncertain. It could be very scary for them. Just let it go.

Who needs it, anyway?

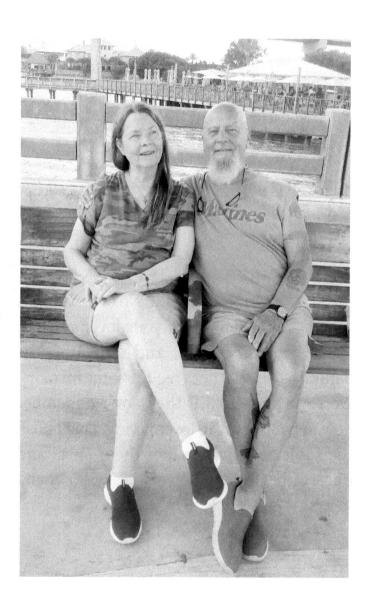

# *Affection*

As a caregiver, your life has changed. When you first met, you were in love. Over the years a lot of things have been taken for granted. You're used to each other and can anticipate each other's moves and thoughts. Now that you're a caregiver, your life has changed more than you would think. Caregiving now has become a job, and with this job it is your priority to take care of your loved one, making sure they are safe, clean, and well fed.

What gets put to the side is the affection you once had. Your loved one still needs to have that affection you would have once given her all the time. Don't forget to hold her hand, give her a kiss, a hug; run your fingers through her hair. Let her know she is still your sweetheart. It makes such a difference to them. They need to know you love them, no matter what.

# Makeup

So let's talk a bit about makeup. Generally speaking, this is mostly for the men taking care of their female loved ones, but let's just say for anyone who likes to have makeup on. I have had a lot of comments from people when they find out that I do my wife's makeup and hair. So I am writing this because I have covered most things that I do; now I am covering the subject of makeup.

Today I came across a professional caregiver. (I am only a semi-pro!) We were talking and she said that my wife didn't look her age. Joking, I said, "It's because I do such a good job putting on her makeup." The caregiver looked at me like I was kidding. I assured her that I wasn't. Then it dawned on me that I should mention this in the book.

Your loved one has probably been wearing makeup most of their life. It always makes them feel good, more presentable, and self-confident. Because they are now at the point that they can't put it on themselves doesn't mean they have to go out with a naked face. Make them feel pretty! Put that makeup on for them.

Might I suggest going to the makeup counter at your local department store.

Talk to the salesperson behind the counter. Explain your situation and ask for a simple way to apply makeup (something you can remember and as few steps as possible).

I have a three-step routine:

1. makeup base;
2. the makeup itself;
3. a good powder.

You want to keep your loved one happy. It's all about being happy!
    An added note:
        Get a good lipstick.
        Don't forget the earrings.
Both are very important. Your loved one will love you for it!

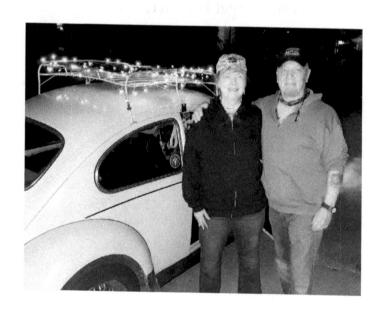

# Music

Let me start off by asking you a question: Did you know that one of the last things to leave an Alzheimer's patient is music? Music has been such a large part of my wife's care. I had three cars at one time and put Sirius Satellite Radio in all three.

One car was a 1970 VW Bug. We bought that car because she could remember when she used to have a Bug. It was just a fun car for her. We put a roof rack on it and decorated it with Christmas lights. The rest of the time we had a surfboard mounted to the roof. After I put the Sirius Radio in, it was an amazing thing! She would sing from the time she sat in the car to the time she got out. She loved listening to songs from the '50s and '60s, the Love channel, and a bit of country. The amazing thing is that she could remember ALL the words! As time went by and her memory went downhill, she didn't even know what car we were in. They all had Sirius Radio, so it made no difference to her. She would just sing! Eventually I sold the VW because she appeared to be getting a little uncomfortable in it.

She doesn't even know that it's missing. She can't make sentences anymore and can't find words for conversation. But when the radio is on, she sings and makes no mistakes. It's wonderful to see her so happy.

It's music to my ears.

What a blessing music can be!

# The Ongoing Conversation

This is my main approach to caregiving. I believe it works for me and my wife. I would like everyone to try it, and maybe it will work for you also. I know some people would rather avoid it, but give it a try. What will it hurt? The conversation my wife and I have always had was a "no secrets" relationship. After she started showing signs of dementia or Alzheimer's, we went to all the doctors and had all the testing done to get a proper diagnosis. She was diagnosed with Alzheimer's. From that point on, we had an ongoing conversation. I would explain to her why things were different, why she would forget things.

Every time something else was lost in her memory, I would sit her down and explain to her that she had Alzheimer's—that she was going to forget more as time went on, but as that happened, I would be there to FILL IN THE BLANKS that she couldn't remember. This conversation would always make her feel better and more relaxed.

Every time something would happen to her memory and she couldn't remember something, or she would show signs of being upset about why she couldn't remember something, that is when I would have the ongoing conversation. There was no limit to how often or the number of times that we would talk. She would always feel relieved after our conversations, and I always told her that I would be here to FILL IN THE BLANKS.

# So You Think You Want to Take a Trip?

*I* know that you get tired of being around the house. We all do. So you want to take a little excursion. If you are planning to go by yourself, just to get away, there are a number of things to think about: Who are you going to leave your loved one with? Will it be at your home or somewhere else? Is it one of the senior services that will come to your home? I certainly recommend a family member or friend that your loved one will be comfortable with. Leave all contact info: yours, emergency, anything that might pop up, medications.

Remember, your loved one is used to a routine. Anything different may throw them off; then they become scared and confused. Keep your routine simple, and make sure your temporary caregiver knows all about it.

It will always be a chore to try to get away. Your life has changed and you need to accept that your loved one is your priority. Your life will never be the same, and there will be more and more responsibility on you.

If you choose to travel (or run away!), do it in the early stages. As the condition progresses, it will be harder to get away. Your loved one will need you more and more all the time, and your duties will become more and more. Now, if you want both of you to get away, or maybe go to a family function: First remember you are taking them out of their most comfortable and familiar environment. You will get a lot of confusion, questions, and they may very likely be scared. You will need a list of what to take:

- Night-light
- Medications
- Change of clothes
- Makeup
- Hair products
- Contact info (should anything happen to you while you're away)

This is just a short list of things you might think about.

I personally would not take my wife out of her environment, where she would be scared and confused. It's just not worth it to me. I would rather have her content, comfortable, and at ease at home.

I heard of a man who sent his wife (by herself) from the East Coast to California. It was a nonstop flight and the flight crew knew she was an Alzheimer's patient. But what if there had been an emergency stop, unexpected bad weather, or unscheduled crew change? I think it was very selfish of her husband. I couldn't do it. Fortunately, she arrived safely. Thank God for all miracles!

# Routine

*I* have touched on routine before. It should not be overlooked! It is extremely important that once you have established a routine with your loved one, you need to keep it up. It is their comfort zone to be in a routine. By changing it you open up to confusion, and then things go downhill. They will not be sure of what is going on and most likely will become scared—a terrible way for them to be! They don't need to be confused and scared. Keep a routine!

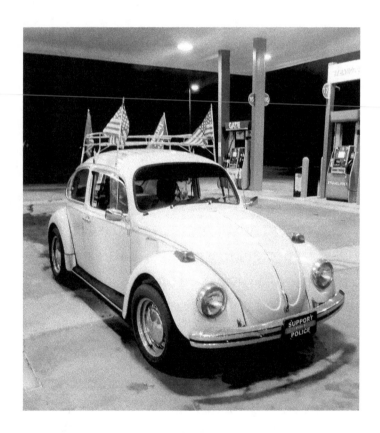

# Driving

O nce they have been diagnosed with dementia, they will start losing their ability to see properly. Their peripheral vision becomes diminished and they lose their depth perception.

Between vision problems and the fact that, in time, they will not be able to follow directions, driving becomes dangerous. They may get lost or be involved in a serious accident. You could even be sued.

Start as early as possible to have them surrender their license. Sometimes it is very difficult to get them to cooperate, and you may need to involve their doctor. Nobody wants to give up their driver's license and their independence!

# Confrontation

Some people with Alzheimer's will sometimes be confrontational. When this happens, you want to remember not to disagree with them. They will only get more determined to be right.

I found that the best way to handle it is to agree with them. They will always be right. The other thing to do is change the subject.

Never argue. It only makes the situation extremely worse.

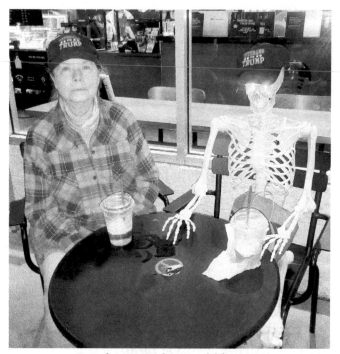

Drink up, or this could be you!

# Dehydration

Boy, can this cause a lot of problems! Keep them well hydrated.

Some people don't like drinking plain water. Try other options, like flavored water, Gatorade, or fruit juices. Just make sure you keep them well hydrated. Dehydration can cause them to become more confused and lightheaded, among other symptoms, and they are at a greater risk of falling. In extreme cases they might have to be admitted to the hospital.

Please keep them well hydrated!

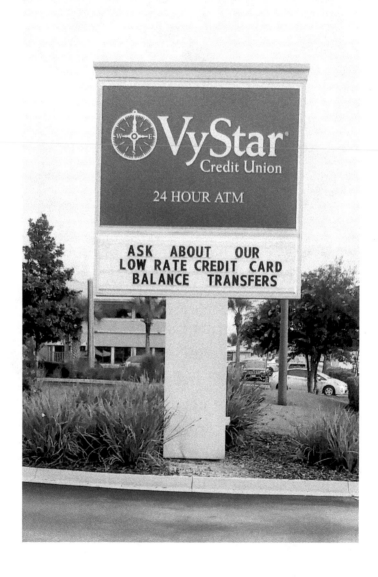

# High Finance and the Future

In many relationships, the finances are handled by only one person. When that person has become the one who needs the care, watch out! Because the other person has no clue what to do. How do you make deposits and withdrawals at the bank? How about moving money from one account to another? Paying bills? Insurances: life, auto, health? Do you have a joint account for all your banking? Do you have access to the funds you may need to care for your partner? Those and many more are questions you need to ask yourself. You need to know and learn all these things early on, before the panic sets in.

What happens to your loved one if something happens to you? Who will take care of your loved one? You need to ask yourself these questions and make the necessary changes. Every situation is a little different. You might want to set up a trust to take care of your finances and future. Find out what your options are.

I know everything is overwhelming! If you have the opportunity to discuss options with your loved one, do it early on, so you are confident and not taken by surprise. If a nursing home may be in your future, look early so you have time to plan options for the future and what would best suit your loved one.

It's a lot to think about, but necessary. Good luck!

# Mourning

Just a little note on mourning: What many people don't realize is that when a person has come down with a life-threatening disease like cancer, Alzheimer's, and many more, the mourning process starts almost immediately. It continues till your loved one is gone. You start missing the things you did together. Little by little, more and more things become missing. Your life has changed and you start noticing that life is not like it used to be. You realize how much things have changed and are not coming back. It's all about mourning. You are grieving each time something else is missing. You want it not to change. But it does, and all you can do is miss all those things you shared.

All this adds up to mourning. It's not like an accident that suddenly takes your loved one away, and then you start mourning.

Feel blessed you have the opportunity to mourn with them while they are still alive.

# The Doctor

I certainly did not want to pass up the doctor.

Hopefully, you will find a doctor you will have a good relationship with. This is so important. Find one who will listen to you and give you the time to hear your concerns. My doctor is a blessing to both of us. He will take as much time as needed to listen to whatever I have to say. He doesn't pretend to know everything and is open to suggestions. He even makes himself available to me after office hours. He knows I need his support.

He has become more than a doctor to us; he is our friend.

I hope you can find a kind, understanding doctor and friend, as we have.

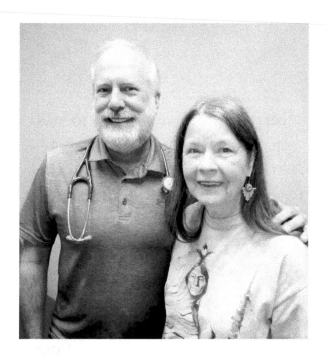

# My Thoughts on Caregiving

*I* have known people who have left their loved one because their loved one was diagnosed with a disease. One person I know—when he found out that his wife had breast cancer, he just picked up and left. I guess he was in that marriage for the good, and not the bad.

I have found all my strength in my faith with the Lord.

I feel I have been chosen to be a caregiver for my loved ones.

What a blessing it is to know you have been picked to take care of someone. When you're in doubt about how to handle a problem or a situation? By praying about it, the answer somehow comes and you now know what to do.

I would not know how to get through a day without my faith.

Yes, I feel blessed and confident as I take care of my loved one, knowing that the Lord is with me.

# Care for the Caregiver

We covered caregiving. Now let's talk about the caregiver.

As the caregiver, you will be subjected to a lot of stress, trying to make all the right decisions—something you had never planned on doing. You always felt that any decisions in your relationship would be something you could discuss together.

Well, here you are, and it's all up to you.

Stress will take its toll. It affects you in ways you aren't aware of. It can destroy your health, raise your blood pressure, cause all kinds of aches and pains, and it will cause you many sleepless nights.

So now we know what stress can do. How do you handle it? Don't keep everything in. Share your concerns with other people. Look for ways you can get a break from caregiving. A couple of days away from your duties. Exercise, meditation. Have someone come in to help you. Don't forget about hospice. Check with them. They're not like the old-time hospice.

People will tell you, "You need to take care of yourself." People mean well, but they're not in your shoes. They don't realize it's not so easy to just take a break from things. If you think about it, you don't need to be told what to do. You know you need to take care of yourself. Bottom line is you need to be well so you can take care of your loved one.

Personally, my faith and prayers have worked for me.

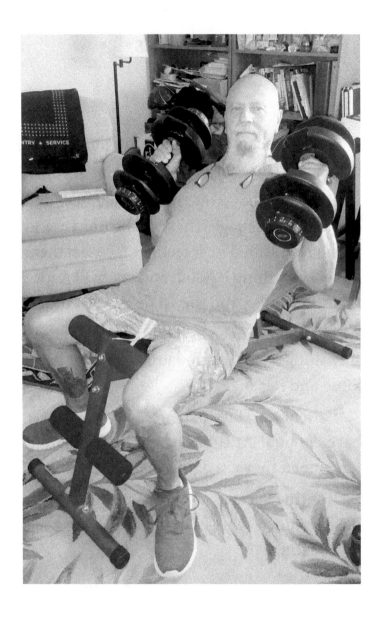

# Key Words

**Acceptance** – Things are not going to get better. Learn to accept and go with the changes.

**Reassurance** – You can read their face and their body language. They will be uneasy and may have a scared look on their face. Let them know everything is good, and you will notice their body relax and they'll be more at peace.

**Laughter** – Keep everything light and do silly things! Have them laugh! It keeps them loose and relaxed.

**Patience** – Have patience. You can never have enough! At times it will be trying, but remember, they are doing the best they can.

**Routine** – Have a routine and stick with it! NO sudden changes in their life helps keep them calm.

# Your Little Worksheet

Ask yourself and fill in the answer:

Acceptance: Have you accepted your situation?


Reassurance: Can you calmly reassure?


Laughter: Can you be silly enough to make them relax and laugh


Patience: Do you need more?


Routine: Can you develop a routine and stick to it?

# Contacts That May Help You

St. Johns County Council on Aging,
St. Augustine, FL: 904-209-3700

Alzheimer's Association:
(24/7 Helpline) 800-272-3900

American Cancer Society:
800-227-2345

St. Jude for Children:
866-278-5833

Shriners Hospitals for Children:
800-237-5055

Google your local Council on Aging;
many offer help.

# Songs That May Help You

Two songs that mean a lot to me; they just open your heart!:

Kathy Mattea – "Where've You Been?"

Collin Raye – "If You Get There Before I Do"

# I Still Remember You
by Jim Hatcher

I know the one I love so much
Yet dwells behind those eyes.
I hear your heart, I feel your touch.
Your life is in disguise.

Your recent memories are few,
You can't recall my name.
But I still reminisce with you,
And love you just the same.

And in some ways my memories
Are stronger than before.
Ironically, that dreaded disease
Helps my heart focus more.

You've loved and lived so faithfully;
Now I will see you through.
For though you don't remember me,
I still remember you.

This page is dedicated to my wife's best friend, Ellen. Better than any sister could be.

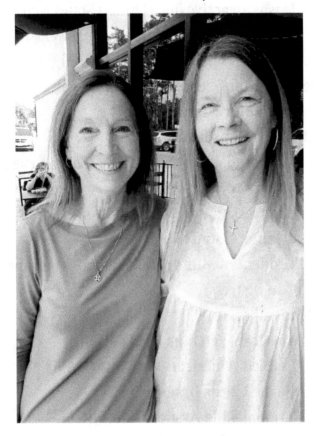

Always full of love, my friend and favorite typist. She is always on call and there when we need her. May she always be blessed.

## Who Is Steve, to Write a Book?

He was an active duty United States Marine. He served four years, 13 months of it fighting in Vietnam. After that, he became a firefighter and fire captain for 26 years. Later, he volunteered for Habitat for Humanity.

**Other positions held:**

Commandant of the Marine Corps League

Commander of the DAV

Vice president of Veterans Council of St. Johns County

President of Vets 4 Vets (help for veterans in distress)

**Life member:**

American Veterans (AMVETS)

Disabled American Veterans (DAV)

Marine Corps League

National Rifle Association (NRA)

Veterans of Foreign Wars (VFW).

As you can see, he has no qualifications to write a book!

## Last Page

Well, I hope you read the whole book and didn't just skip to the last page! I hope that you can take something from the book and maybe you can make some small changes to the things I have mentioned, and, hopefully, it will make your life a little easier.

All proceeds from this book
will be split between:

**the Alzheimer's Foundation**
and
**the American Cancer Society.**

CPSIA information can be obtained
at www.ICGtesting.com
Printed in the USA
LVHW022026300323
743062LV00002B/301